MALE FERTILITY COOKBOOK

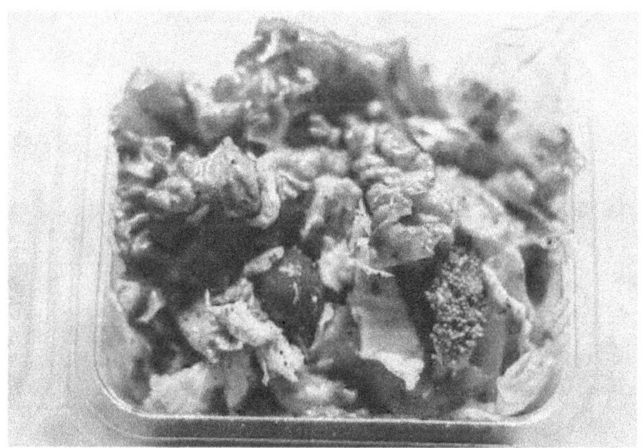

DR. JESSICA SMITH

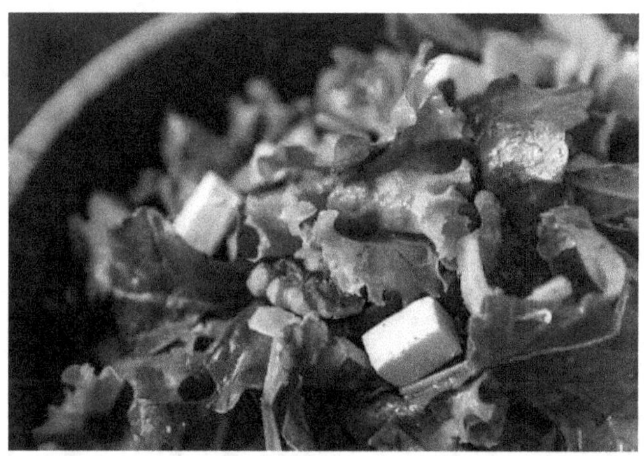

TABLE OF CONTENTS

CHAPTER ONE

How to Use this Cookbook

Introduction and Familiarization:

Begin by familiarizing yourself with the Male Fertility Cookbook. Read the introduction to understand the cookbook's purpose, the importance of nutrition for male fertility, and the overall approach to enhancing reproductive health through diet.

Ingredient Preparation:

Review the list of ingredients commonly used in the recipes. Ensure your kitchen is stocked with key items such as fertility-boosting foods, vitamins, and minerals. This may include fruits, vegetables, lean proteins, whole grains, and specific fertility-promoting nutrients.

Meal Planning:

Plan your meals according to the cookbook's suggested recipes. Consider incorporating a variety of dishes that encompass different nutrients and flavors to keep your diet diverse and enjoyable.

Understanding Nutrient-Rich Foods:

Pay attention to the nutritional benefits of the ingredients used. The cookbook likely highlights foods rich in antioxidants, vitamins, and minerals known to support male fertility. Familiarize yourself with the specific nutrients that contribute to reproductive health.

Portion Control:

Follow recommended portion sizes outlined in the cookbook. Maintaining appropriate portion control is essential for a balanced diet and optimal fertility. Overeating or undereating can impact overall health and potentially affect fertility.

Meal Timing:

Pay attention to meal timing. The cookbook may suggest optimal times for meals and snacks to ensure a steady supply of nutrients throughout the day. Consistency in eating patterns can positively influence fertility.

Hydration:

Stay hydrated. Adequate water intake is crucial for overall health and can support reproductive functions. The cookbook may offer suggestions for hydrating beverages that complement fertility goals.

Cooking Techniques:

Learn and practice cooking techniques recommended in the cookbook. Understanding how to prepare meals using methods that preserve nutritional value is essential for maximizing the benefits of fertility-boosting ingredients.

Supplement Integration:

If the cookbook suggests specific supplements to complement the recipes, consider integrating them into your routine. Always consult with a healthcare professional before adding new supplements to your diet.

Monitoring Progress:

Pay attention to how your body responds to the dietary changes. Monitor energy levels, overall well-being, and any improvements in reproductive health. If necessary, consult a healthcare professional for personalized advice on optimizing male fertility.

Understanding male fertility involves recognizing the intricate biological processes that contribute to reproductive health in men.

Male fertility hinges on the successful production, maturation, and delivery of healthy sperm. The testes, located within the scrotum, are central to this process, producing sperm and testosterone.

Several factors influence male fertility, including sperm count, motility, and morphology.

Sperm count refers to the number of sperm in a given sample, while motility indicates their ability to move effectively. Morphology assesses the shape and structure of sperm, crucial for successful fertilization.

Lifestyle factors play a pivotal role in male fertility. A balanced diet rich in essential nutrients, regular exercise, and the avoidance of harmful habits such as smoking and excessive alcohol consumption contribute to optimal reproductive health.

Stress management is also crucial, as chronic stress can adversely affect fertility.

Various medical conditions, hormonal imbalances, genetic factors, and environmental exposures can impact male fertility.

Seeking professional guidance, particularly from a reproductive endocrinologist or urologist, can aid in understanding and addressing fertility challenges.

Comprehensive understanding involves acknowledging that male fertility is dynamic, influenced by a multitude of factors, and can be optimized through a holistic approach encompassing lifestyle modifications, proper nutrition, and informed medical care.

Cultivating this awareness is essential for those navigating the journey toward parenthood and seeking to foster reproductive well-being.

Principles of Male Fertility

The principles of male fertility revolve around maintaining a conducive environment for the optimal function of the male reproductive system.

Key principles include:

Sperm Production and Quality:

The foundation of male fertility lies in the continuous production of healthy sperm. Spermatogenesis, the process occurring in the testes, must proceed efficiently for high-quality sperm to be available for fertilization.

Hormonal Balance:

Hormones play a pivotal role in male fertility, with testosterone being a primary regulator. Maintaining a delicate balance of hormones is crucial for supporting sperm production, sexual function, and overall reproductive health.

Nutrient-Rich Diet:

A well-balanced and nutrient-rich diet is fundamental to male fertility. Essential vitamins and minerals, such as zinc, selenium, and antioxidants, contribute to sperm quality and protect reproductive cells from oxidative stress.

Lifestyle Factors:

Healthy lifestyle choices positively impact male fertility. Regular exercise, abstaining from smoking, limiting alcohol intake, and managing stress are essential principles. Unhealthy habits can disrupt hormonal balance and impair sperm production.

Temperature Regulation:

The testes function optimally at a slightly lower temperature than the rest of the body. Principles of male fertility include practices that avoid excessive heat, such as avoiding hot baths, saunas, or prolonged exposure to heated environments.

Regular Sexual Activity:

Regular sexual activity supports sperm health by preventing the accumulation of DNA damage and promoting sperm motility. Maintaining a consistent sexual routine contributes to reproductive well-being.

Medical Checkups:

Regular medical checkups with a healthcare professional or urologist are essential. Monitoring reproductive health allows for the early detection and management of any potential issues affecting fertility.

Benefits of Male Fertility

The benefits of optimal male fertility extend beyond the realm of procreation, influencing overall well-being and contributing to a man's holistic health.

Successful Reproduction:

The primary benefit is, of course, the ability to successfully conceive and contribute to the creation of a family. Healthy sperm, characterized by adequate count, motility, and morphology, enhances the chances of fertilization.

Enhanced Sexual Health:

Male fertility is closely linked to sexual health. Maintaining reproductive function supports libido, erectile function, and overall sexual satisfaction, contributing to a fulfilling intimate life.

Psychological Well-being:

The ability to conceive can positively impact a man's mental and emotional state. Successful reproduction often brings a sense of fulfillment, boosting self-esteem and confidence.

Holistic Health: Practices that support male fertility, such as maintaining a balanced diet, regular exercise, and avoiding harmful habits, contribute to overall health. These habits can help prevent or manage conditions such as obesity, diabetes, and cardiovascular issues.

Long-Term Relationship Satisfaction:

Successfully conceiving and starting a family can enhance long-term relationship satisfaction. The shared experience of parenthood often strengthens emotional bonds and fosters a sense of partnership. .

Generational Legacy:

The ability to pass on one's genetic material to future generations is a profound benefit of male fertility. Contributing to the creation of a family establishes a generational legacy and can bring a sense of continuity and connection.

Recognizing and nurturing male fertility not only supports the desire for offspring but also lays the foundation for a healthier, more fulfilling life. Embracing habits that enhance reproductive health is a proactive investment in both present well-being and the potential for a thriving future.

Optimizing male fertility involves incorporating lifestyle choices and practices that support reproductive health. Here are key tips for promoting male fertility:

Balanced Nutrition:

Maintain a well-balanced diet rich in essential nutrients. Incorporate foods high in antioxidants, such as fruits, vegetables, nuts, and seeds, to support sperm health and protect against oxidative stress.

Hydration:

Stay adequately hydrated as water is essential for overall health, including reproductive functions. Proper hydration ensures the optimal production and transport of sperm.

Maintain a Healthy Weight: Strive for a healthy weight through regular exercise and a balanced diet. Obesity or underweight conditions can impact hormonal balance and sperm production.

Limit Alcohol and Quit Smoking:

Reduce alcohol consumption and quit smoking. Both habits can negatively affect sperm quality and reproductive health.

Moderate Exercise:

Engage in regular, moderate-intensity exercise. Physical activity contributes to overall health and can positively impact reproductive functions. However, excessive exercise may have adverse effects, so moderation is key.

Stress Management:

Practice stress-reducing techniques such as meditation, yoga, or deep breathing. Chronic stress can impact hormonal balance and reproductive health.

Avoid Overheating:

Avoid prolonged exposure to high temperatures, such as hot baths, saunas, or tight-fitting underwear. Elevated testicular temperature can affect sperm production.

Regular Sexual Activity: Maintain a regular sexual activity routine. Frequent ejaculation can prevent the accumulation of DNA damage in sperm and support overall reproductive health.

Limit Exposure to Toxins: Be mindful of exposure to environmental toxins, pesticides, and pollutants that can negatively impact sperm quality. Take precautions in occupational settings with potential hazards.

Regular Checkups:

Schedule regular checkups with a healthcare professional or urologist to monitor reproductive health. Early detection and management of potential issues can positively impact fertility.

Guidelines for Male Fertility

Guidelines for optimizing male fertility encompass a holistic approach that addresses various aspects of lifestyle, nutrition, and healthcare:

Regular Checkups: Schedule routine checkups with a healthcare professional or urologist to monitor reproductive health. Regular assessments can detect potential issues early and facilitate timely intervention.

Healthy Lifestyle Habits:

Cultivate healthy lifestyle habits, including regular exercise, a balanced diet, and adequate sleep. These practices contribute to overall well-being and support optimal reproductive functions.

Balanced Diet:

Embrace a nutrient-rich and well-balanced diet. Prioritize foods rich in antioxidants, vitamins, and minerals, which are essential for sperm health. Consider supplements if necessary, consulting with a healthcare professional for guidance.

Maintain a Healthy Weight:

Strive for a healthy weight through a combination of regular physical activity and a nutritious diet. Excess weight or being underweight can impact hormonal balance and fertility.

Limit Environmental Exposures: Minimize exposure to environmental toxins, pollutants, and potentially harmful substances. Be mindful of occupational hazards and take precautions to protect reproductive health.

Manage Stress:

Implement stress-management techniques, such as meditation, yoga, or mindfulness. Chronic stress can adversely affect hormonal balance and reproductive functions.

Avoid Smoking and Excessive Alcohol:

Quit smoking and limit alcohol consumption. Both habits can negatively impact sperm quality and overall reproductive health.

Limit Caffeine Intake:

Moderate caffeine intake. While the evidence on caffeine's direct impact is inconclusive, excessive consumption may affect fertility in some individuals.

Regular Sexual Activity:

Maintain a regular and healthy sexual activity routine. Frequent ejaculation can prevent sperm stagnation and support overall reproductive health.

Seek Professional Advice:

If experiencing fertility challenges, seek guidance from fertility specialists. Consulting with a reproductive endocrinologist or urologist can provide personalized recommendations and potential fertility treatments.

CHAPTER TWO

1: Fertility-Boosting Smoothie Bowl

Ingredients:

- 1 cup mixed berries (blueberries, strawberries, raspberries)
- 1 banana
- 1/2 cup Greek yogurt
- 1 tablespoon chia seeds
- 1 tablespoon pumpkin seeds
- 1 tablespoon honey
- 1/2 cup almond milk

Instructions:

- Blend mixed berries, banana, Greek yogurt, chia seeds, pumpkin seeds, honey, and almond milk until smooth.
- Pour the smoothie into a bowl.
- Top with additional berries, chia seeds, and pumpkin seeds.
- Enjoy this nutrient-packed smoothie bowl.

Health Benefits:

- ➢ Berries are rich in antioxidants.
- ➢ Chia seeds and pumpkin seeds provide essential nutrients for reproductive health.
- ➢ Greek yogurt contributes to probiotics and protein.

Preparation Time: 10 minutes

2: Quinoa and Salmon Power Bowl

Ingredients:

- ➢ 1 cup cooked quinoa
- ➢ 4 oz grilled salmon
- ➢ 1 cup steamed broccoli
- ➢ 1/2 avocado, sliced
- ➢ 1 tablespoon olive oil
- ➢ Lemon juice, salt, and pepper to taste

Instructions:

- ➢ Arrange cooked quinoa as the base in a bowl.
- ➢ Top with grilled salmon, steamed broccoli, and sliced avocado.
- ➢ Drizzle with olive oil and lemon juice.
- ➢ Season with salt and pepper to taste.

> Mix and enjoy this nutrient-dense power bowl.

Health Benefits:

> Quinoa provides protein and essential amino acids.

> Salmon offers omega-3 fatty acids for sperm health.

> Broccoli and avocado contribute vitamins and minerals.

Preparation Time: 20 minutes

3: Spinach and Walnut Salad

Ingredients:

> 2 cups fresh spinach

> 1/2 cup cherry tomatoes, halved

> 1/4 cup feta cheese, crumbled

> 1/4 cup walnuts, chopped

> 1 tablespoon olive oil

> Balsamic vinegar, salt, and pepper to taste

Instructions:

> In a bowl, combine fresh spinach, cherry tomatoes, feta cheese, and walnuts.

> Drizzle with olive oil and balsamic vinegar.

> Season with salt and pepper to taste.

> Toss well and serve this nutritious salad.

Health Benefits:

> Spinach is rich in folate, a crucial nutrient for male fertility.
> Walnuts provide omega-3 fatty acids.
> Feta cheese adds protein and calcium.

Preparation Time: 15 minutes

4: Lentil and Vegetable Stew

Ingredients:

> 1 cup dried green lentils (rinsed)
> 2 carrots, chopped
> 2 celery stalks, chopped
> 1 onion, diced
> 3 cloves garlic, minced
> 4 cups vegetable broth
> 1 teaspoon cumin
> 1 teaspoon turmeric
> Salt and pepper to taste

Instructions:

- In a pot, sauté onions and garlic until translucent.
- Add lentils, carrots, celery, cumin, turmeric, salt, and pepper.
- Pour in vegetable broth and bring to a boil.
- Simmer until lentils and vegetables are tender.
- Serve this hearty stew warm.

Health Benefits:

- Lentils are high in protein and folate.
- Vegetables provide essential vitamins and minerals.
- Turmeric has anti-inflammatory properties.

Preparation Time: 30 minutes

5: Berry and Nut Yogurt Parfait

Ingredients:

- 1 cup Greek yogurt
- 1/2 cup granola
- 1/2 cup mixed berries (strawberries, blueberries)
- 2 tablespoons almonds, sliced
- 1 tablespoon honey

Instructions:

- ➢ In a glass or bowl, layer Greek yogurt, granola, mixed berries, and sliced almonds.
- ➢ Repeat the layers.
- ➢ Drizzle honey over the top.
- ➢ Enjoy this delicious and fertility-boosting parfait.

Health Benefits:

- ➢ Greek yogurt provides probiotics and protein.
- ➢ Berries offer antioxidants.
- ➢ Almonds contribute healthy fats and vitamin E.

Preparation Time: 10 minutes

6: Shrimp and Asparagus Stir-Fry

Ingredients:

- ➢ 8 oz shrimp, peeled and deveined
- ➢ 1 bunch asparagus, trimmed and cut into bite-sized pieces
- ➢ 2 cloves garlic, minced
- ➢ 1 tablespoon ginger, grated
- ➢ 2 tablespoons soy sauce (low-sodium)
- ➢ 1 tablespoon olive oil

> Brown rice for serving

Instructions:

> In a pan, heat olive oil and sauté garlic and ginger until fragrant.
> Add shrimp and cook until pink.
> Add asparagus and soy sauce, stir-fry until asparagus is tender.
> Serve over brown rice.

Health Benefits:

> Shrimp provides lean protein.
> Asparagus is rich in vitamins and antioxidants.
> Garlic and ginger have anti-inflammatory properties.

Preparation Time: 15 minutes

7: Sweet Potato and Black Bean Bowl

Ingredients:

> 1 medium sweet potato, cubed
> 1 can black beans, drained and rinsed
> 1 cup corn kernels (fresh or frozen)
> 1 teaspoon cumin
> 1 teaspoon chili powder

- ➢ 2 tablespoons olive oil
- ➢ Fresh cilantro for garnish

Instructions:

- ➢ Toss sweet potato cubes with olive oil, cumin, and chili powder.
- ➢ Roast in the oven until tender.
- ➢ In a bowl, combine roasted sweet potato, black beans, and corn.
- ➢ Garnish with fresh cilantro.

Health Benefits:

- ➢ Sweet potatoes offer vitamins and fiber.
- ➢ Black beans provide protein and folate.
- ➢ Corn adds fiber and antioxidants.

Preparation Time: 25 minutes

8: Pumpkin Seed and Spinach Pesto Pasta

Ingredients:

- ➢ 8 oz whole grain or lentil pasta
- ➢ 2 cups fresh spinach
- ➢ 1/2 cup pumpkin seeds (pepitas)
- ➢ 2 cloves garlic

- ➢ 1/4 cup nutritional yeast

- ➢ 1/4 cup olive oil

- ➢ Lemon juice, salt, and pepper to taste

Instructions:

- ➢ Cook pasta according to package instructions.

- ➢ In a food processor, blend spinach, pumpkin seeds, garlic, nutritional yeast, olive oil, lemon juice, salt, and pepper until smooth.

- ➢ Toss the pesto with cooked pasta.

- ➢ Serve with a sprinkle of nutritional yeast.

Health Benefits:

- ➢ Whole grain pasta provides fiber.

- ➢ Spinach is rich in iron and folate.

- ➢ Pumpkin seeds offer zinc and healthy fats.

Preparation Time: 20 minutes

9: Chicken and Quinoa Salad

Ingredients:

- ➢ 1 cup cooked quinoa

- ➢ 1 cup grilled chicken breast, sliced

- ➢ 1 cup cherry tomatoes, halved

- ➢ 1 cucumber, diced
- ➢ 1/4 cup feta cheese, crumbled
- ➢ 2 tablespoons balsamic vinaigrette dressing

Instructions:

- ➢ In a bowl, combine cooked quinoa, grilled chicken, cherry tomatoes, cucumber, and feta cheese.
- ➢ Drizzle with balsamic vinaigrette dressing.
- ➢ Toss gently to combine.
- ➢ Enjoy this protein-packed salad.

Health Benefits:

- ➢ Quinoa provides complete protein.
- ➢ Grilled chicken offers lean protein.
- ➢ Vegetables contribute vitamins and minerals.

Preparation Time: 15 minutes

10: Mango and Avocado Salsa with Grilled Fish

Ingredients:

- ➢ 2 fish fillets (such as tilapia or cod)
- ➢ 1 ripe mango, diced

- 1 avocado, diced
- 1/4 cup red onion, finely chopped
- 1/4 cup cilantro, chopped
- Lime juice, salt, and pepper to taste

Instructions:

- Grill fish fillets until cooked through.
- In a bowl, combine diced mango, avocado, red onion, cilantro, lime juice, salt, and pepper.
- Serve the grilled fish topped with mango and avocado salsa.

Health Benefits:

- Fish provides omega-3 fatty acids.
- Mango and avocado offer vitamins and healthy fats.
- Cilantro adds antioxidants.

Preparation Time: 20 minutes

11: Broccoli and Turkey Quiche

Ingredients:

- 1 pie crust (whole wheat or alternative)
- 1 cup broccoli florets, steamed
- 1/2 lb ground turkey, cooked

- ➢ 1 cup shredded cheddar cheese
- ➢ 4 large eggs
- ➢ 1 cup milk (dairy or plant-based)
- ➢ Salt and pepper to taste

Instructions:

- ➢ Preheat the oven and bake the pie crust according to package instructions.
- ➢ Layer cooked ground turkey, steamed broccoli, and shredded cheddar cheese in the pie crust.
- ➢ In a bowl, whisk together eggs, milk, salt, and pepper.
- ➢ Pour the egg mixture over the ingredients in the pie crust.
- ➢ Bake until the quiche is set and golden brown.

Health Benefits:

- ➢ Broccoli provides folate and fiber.
- ➢ Turkey offers lean protein.
- ➢ Eggs supply essential vitamins and minerals.

Preparation Time: 45 minutes

12: Cauliflower and Chickpea Curry

Ingredients:

> * 1 cauliflower, cut into florets
> * 1 can chickpeas, drained and rinsed
> * 1 onion, finely chopped
> * 2 cloves garlic, minced
> * 1 can coconut milk
> * 2 tablespoons curry powder
> * 1 tablespoon olive oil
> * Basmati rice for serving

Instructions:

> * In a pot, sauté onions and garlic in olive oil until softened.
> * Add cauliflower, chickpeas, curry powder, and coconut milk.
> * Simmer until cauliflower is tender.
> * Serve the curry over cooked basmati rice.

Health Benefits:

> * Cauliflower provides vitamins C and K.
> * Chickpeas offer protein and fiber.

> Coconut milk adds healthy fats.

Preparation Time: 30 minutes

13: Blueberry and Almond Overnight Oats

Ingredients:

- 1/2 cup rolled oats
- 1/2 cup almond milk
- 1/4 cup Greek yogurt
- 1/2 cup blueberries
- 1 tablespoon almond butter
- 1 teaspoon chia seeds

Instructions:

- In a jar, combine rolled oats, almond milk, Greek yogurt, blueberries, almond butter, and chia seeds.
- Stir well, ensuring oats are fully immersed in liquid.
- Refrigerate overnight.
- In the morning, give it a good stir and enjoy this nutritious breakfast.

Health Benefits:

- Blueberries are rich in antioxidants.
- Almond butter provides healthy fats.

➢ Greek yogurt adds protein and probiotics.

Preparation Time: 10 minutes (plus overnight refrigeration)

14: Grilled Vegetable and Quinoa Stuffed Bell Peppers

Ingredients:

- ➢ 4 bell peppers, halved
- ➢ 1 cup cooked quinoa
- ➢ 1 zucchini, diced
- ➢ 1 yellow squash, diced
- ➢ 1 cup cherry tomatoes, halved
- ➢ 1/2 cup feta cheese, crumbled
- ➢ 2 tablespoons olive oil
- ➢ Italian seasoning, salt, and pepper to taste

Instructions:

- ➢ Preheat the grill.
- ➢ In a bowl, mix cooked quinoa, diced zucchini, yellow squash, cherry tomatoes, feta cheese, olive oil, Italian seasoning, salt, and pepper.
- ➢ Fill each bell pepper half with the quinoa mixture.
- ➢ Grill until the peppers are tender.

Health Benefits:

> Quinoa provides protein and fiber.
> Grilled vegetables offer vitamins and antioxidants.
> Feta cheese adds calcium and flavor.

Preparation Time: 25 minutes

15: Pistachio-Crusted Salmon

Ingredients:

> 2 salmon fillets
> 1/2 cup pistachios, crushed
> 1 tablespoon Dijon mustard
> 1 tablespoon honey
> Lemon wedges for serving

Instructions:

> Preheat the oven.
> Mix crushed pistachios, Dijon mustard, and honey in a bowl.
> Coat the salmon fillets with the pistachio mixture.
> Bake until the salmon is cooked through.
> Serve with lemon wedges.

Health Benefits:

- ➢ Salmon provides omega-3 fatty acids.
- ➢ Pistachios offer protein and healthy fats.
- ➢ Honey adds natural sweetness.

Preparation Time: 20 minutes

16: Turkey and Vegetable Stir-Fry with Brown Rice

Ingredients:

- ➢ 1 lb ground turkey
- ➢ 2 cups mixed vegetables (broccoli, bell peppers, snap peas)
- ➢ 2 tablespoons soy sauce (low-sodium)
- ➢ 1 tablespoon sesame oil
- ➢ 1 tablespoon ginger, minced
- ➢ 3 cups cooked brown rice

Instructions:

- ➢ In a wok or skillet, cook ground turkey until browned.
- ➢ Add mixed vegetables and ginger, stir-frying until vegetables are tender.

➢ Drizzle with soy sauce and sesame oil, mixing well.

➢ Serve the stir-fry over cooked brown rice.

Health Benefits:

➢ Turkey provides lean protein.

➢ Mixed vegetables offer vitamins and fiber.

➢ Brown rice adds complex carbohydrates.

Preparation Time: 25 minutes

17: Berry and Spinach Smoothie

Ingredients:

➢ 1 cup mixed berries (strawberries, blueberries, raspberries)

➢ 2 cups fresh spinach

➢ 1 banana

➢ 1 cup almond milk

➢ 1 tablespoon flaxseeds

➢ 1 tablespoon honey

Instructions:

➢ Blend mixed berries, fresh spinach, banana, almond milk, flaxseeds, and honey until smooth.

> Pour into a glass and enjoy this nutrient-packed smoothie.

Health Benefits:

> Berries provide antioxidants.

> Spinach is rich in folate and iron.

> Flaxseeds offer omega-3 fatty acids.

Preparation Time: 10 minutes

18: Lentil and Vegetable Curry

Ingredients:

> 1 cup dried red lentils (rinsed)

> 1 sweet potato, diced

> 1 can diced tomatoes

> 1 can coconut milk

> 1 onion, finely chopped

> 2 cloves garlic, minced

> 2 tablespoons curry powder

> Fresh cilantro for garnish

Instructions:

> In a pot, sauté onions and garlic until softened.

- Add dried red lentils, sweet potato, diced tomatoes, coconut milk, and curry powder.
- Simmer until lentils and sweet potato are cooked.
- Garnish with fresh cilantro and serve.

Health Benefits:

- Red lentils provide protein and fiber.
- Sweet potatoes offer vitamins and antioxidants.
- Coconut milk adds healthy fats.

Preparation Time: 30 minutes

19: Avocado and Chickpea Salad

Ingredients:

- 2 avocados, diced
- 1 can chickpeas, drained and rinsed
- 1 cucumber, diced
- 1/4 cup red onion, finely chopped
- 2 tablespoons olive oil
- Lemon juice, salt, and pepper to taste

Instructions:

- In a bowl, combine diced avocados, chickpeas, cucumber, and red onion.

- ➤ Drizzle with olive oil and lemon juice.
- ➤ Season with salt and pepper to taste.
- ➤ Toss gently and serve this refreshing salad.

Health Benefits:

- ➤ Avocados provide healthy fats and vitamins.
- ➤ Chickpeas offer protein and fiber.
- ➤ Cucumber adds hydration and vitamins.

Preparation Time: 15 minutes

20: Almond-Crusted Chicken with Roasted Vegetables

Ingredients:

- ➤ 2 boneless, skinless chicken breasts
- ➤ 1/2 cup almond meal
- ➤ 1 teaspoon paprika
- ➤ 1 teaspoon garlic powder
- ➤ 1 teaspoon dried thyme
- ➤ Assorted vegetables (carrots, Brussels sprouts, bell peppers)
- ➤ 2 tablespoons olive oil
- ➤ Salt and pepper to taste

Instructions:

> Preheat the oven.

> Mix almond meal, paprika, garlic powder, and dried thyme.

> Coat chicken breasts with the almond mixture.

> Arrange chicken and vegetables on a baking sheet, drizzle with olive oil, and season with salt and pepper.

> Roast until chicken is cooked through and vegetables are tender.

Health Benefits:

> Almond meal provides healthy fats and protein.

> Chicken offers lean protein.

> Vegetables add vitamins and fiber.

Preparation Time: 30 minutes

21: Quinoa and Black Bean Stuffed Peppers

Ingredients:

> 4 bell peppers, halved

> 1 cup cooked quinoa

> 1 can black beans, drained and rinsed

- ➢ 1 cup corn kernels (fresh or frozen)
- ➢ 1 cup salsa
- ➢ 1 teaspoon cumin
- ➢ 1 teaspoon chili powder
- ➢ Shredded cheese for topping

Instructions:

- ➢ Preheat the oven.
- ➢ In a bowl, mix cooked quinoa, black beans, corn, salsa, cumin, and chili powder.
- ➢ Fill each bell pepper half with the quinoa mixture.
- ➢ Top with shredded cheese.
- ➢ Bake until the peppers are tender.

Health Benefits:

- ➢ Quinoa provides complete protein.
- ➢ Black beans offer protein and fiber.
- ➢ Corn adds antioxidants.

Preparation Time: 25 minutes

22: Walnut and Banana Pancakes

Ingredients:

- ➢ 1 cup whole wheat flour

- ➤ 1/2 cup chopped walnuts
- ➤ 1 ripe banana, mashed
- ➤ 1 cup almond milk
- ➤ 1 tablespoon maple syrup
- ➤ 1 teaspoon baking powder
- ➤ Coconut oil for cooking

Instructions:

- ➤ In a bowl, mix whole wheat flour, chopped walnuts, mashed banana, almond milk, maple syrup, and baking powder.
- ➤ Heat coconut oil in a pan.
- ➤ Pour pancake batter onto the pan and cook until bubbles form.
- ➤ Flip and cook the other side.
- ➤ Serve with additional banana slices and a drizzle of maple syrup.

Health Benefits:

- ➤ Whole wheat flour provides fiber.
- ➤ Walnuts offer omega-3 fatty acids.

Banana adds natural sweetness.

Preparation Time: 20 minutes

23: Pomegranate and Spinach Salad with Grilled Chicken

Ingredients:

- ➢ 2 boneless, skinless chicken breasts
- ➢ 4 cups fresh spinach
- ➢ 1 cup pomegranate arils
- ➢ 1/2 cup feta cheese, crumbled
- ➢ 1/4 cup balsamic vinaigrette dressing
- ➢ 1/4 cup walnuts, chopped

Instructions:

- ➢ Grill chicken breasts until cooked through.
- ➢ In a large bowl, combine fresh spinach, pomegranate arils, feta cheese, and walnuts.
- ➢ Slice grilled chicken and place on top of the salad.
- ➢ Drizzle with balsamic vinaigrette dressing.

Health Benefits:

- ➢ Spinach provides iron and folate.
- ➢ Pomegranate offers antioxidants.
- ➢ Walnuts add omega-3 fatty acids.

Preparation Time: 25 minutes

24: Ginger Turmeric Carrot Soup

Ingredients:

- 1 lb carrots, peeled and chopped
- 1 onion, chopped
- 3 cloves garlic, minced
- 1 tablespoon fresh ginger, grated
- 1 teaspoon ground turmeric
- 4 cups vegetable broth
- 1 can coconut milk
- 2 tablespoons olive oil
- Salt and pepper to taste

Instructions:

- In a pot, sauté onions, garlic, and ginger in olive oil until softened.
- Add chopped carrots, ground turmeric, and vegetable broth.
- Simmer until carrots are tender.
- Blend the soup until smooth, then stir in coconut milk.
- Season with salt and pepper.

Health Benefits:

- ➤ Carrots offer beta-carotene and vitamins.
- ➤ Ginger and turmeric have anti-inflammatory properties.
- ➤ Coconut milk adds healthy fats.

Preparation Time: 30 minutes

25: Berry and Greek Yogurt Parfait

Ingredients:

- ➤ 2 cups Greek yogurt
- ➤ 1 cup mixed berries (strawberries, blueberries, raspberries)
- ➤ 1/2 cup granola
- ➤ 1 tablespoon honey
- ➤ Mint leaves for garnish

Instructions:

- ➤ In serving glasses, layer Greek yogurt, mixed berries, and granola.
- ➤ Repeat the layers.
- ➤ Drizzle with honey and garnish with mint leaves.
- ➤ Enjoy this refreshing and protein-packed parfait.

Health Benefits:

> ➢ Greek yogurt provides protein and probiotics.
> ➢ Berries offer antioxidants.
> ➢ Granola adds fiber and crunch.

Preparation Time: 15 minutes

26: Turkey and Sweet Potato Chili

Ingredients:

> ➢ 1 lb ground turkey
> ➢ 2 sweet potatoes, diced
> ➢ 1 can black beans, drained and rinsed
> ➢ 1 can diced tomatoes
> ➢ 1 onion, chopped
> ➢ 2 cloves garlic, minced
> ➢ 2 tablespoons chili powder
> ➢ 1 teaspoon cumin
> ➢ Salt and pepper to taste

Instructions:

> ➢ In a pot, cook ground turkey until browned.
> ➢ Add chopped sweet potatoes, black beans, diced tomatoes, onions, garlic, chili powder, and cumin.

> Simmer until sweet potatoes are tender.

> Season with salt and pepper.

Health Benefits:

> Sweet potatoes provide vitamins and fiber.

> Turkey offers lean protein.

> Black beans add protein and fiber.

Preparation Time: 40 minutes

27: Salmon and Quinoa Bowl with Lemon-Dill Dressing

Ingredients:

> 2 salmon fillets

> 1 cup cooked quinoa

> 1 cucumber, diced

> 1 cup cherry tomatoes, halved

> 1/4 cup red onion, finely chopped

> 2 tablespoons fresh dill, chopped

> Juice of 1 lemon

> Olive oil, salt, and pepper to taste

Instructions:

> ➢ Grill salmon fillets until cooked through.
> ➢ In a bowl, combine cooked quinoa, diced cucumber, cherry tomatoes, and red onion.
> ➢ Whisk together lemon juice, olive oil, salt, and pepper to make the dressing.
> ➢ Place grilled salmon on top of the quinoa mixture and drizzle with lemon-dill dressing.

Health Benefits:

> ➢ Salmon provides omega-3 fatty acids.
> ➢ Quinoa offers complete protein.
> ➢ Vegetables add vitamins and minerals.

Preparation Time: 25 minutes

28: Spinach and Mushroom Omelette

Ingredients:

> ➢ 3 large eggs
> ➢ 1 cup fresh spinach
> ➢ 1/2 cup mushrooms, sliced
> ➢ 1/4 cup feta cheese, crumbled
> ➢ 1 tablespoon olive oil

> Salt and pepper to taste

Instructions:

> In a pan, sauté mushrooms and spinach in olive oil until wilted.
> In a bowl, beat eggs and season with salt and pepper.
> Pour the beaten eggs over the vegetables in the pan.
> Sprinkle crumbled feta cheese on top.
> Cook until the eggs are set, then fold the omelette.

Health Benefits:

> Eggs provide protein and essential nutrients.
> Spinach offers iron and folate.
> Feta cheese adds calcium and flavor.

Preparation Time: 15 minutes

29: Almond and Berry Chia Pudding

Ingredients:

> 1/4 cup chia seeds
> 1 cup almond milk
> 1/2 cup mixed berries (strawberries, blueberries)
> 1/4 cup almonds, sliced
> 1 tablespoon maple syrup

Instructions:

- ➢ In a jar, mix chia seeds and almond milk.
- ➢ Refrigerate for at least 2 hours or overnight.
- ➢ In the morning, layer chia pudding with mixed berries and sliced almonds.
- ➢ Drizzle with maple syrup before serving.

Health Benefits:

- ➢ Chia seeds provide omega-3 fatty acids and fiber.
- ➢ Almond milk offers a dairy-free alternative.
- ➢ Berries add antioxidants.

Preparation Time: 10 minutes (plus chilling time)

30: Grilled Veggie and Hummus Wrap

Ingredients:

- ➢ Whole grain tortillas
- ➢ 1 zucchini, sliced
- ➢ 1 red bell pepper, sliced
- ➢ 1 yellow bell pepper, sliced
- ➢ 1 cup cherry tomatoes, halved
- ➢ 1/2 cup hummus
- ➢ Fresh basil leaves

> Olive oil, salt, and pepper to taste

Instructions:

> Preheat the grill.
> Brush zucchini, bell peppers, and cherry tomatoes with olive oil, then grill until tender.
> Spread hummus on whole grain tortillas.
> Layer grilled vegetables and fresh basil leaves.
> Roll into a wrap and secure with toothpicks if needed.

Health Benefits:

> Whole grain tortillas provide fiber.
> Grilled vegetables offer vitamins and antioxidants.
> Hummus adds plant-based protein.

Preparation Time: 20 minutes

31: Eggplant and Lentil Stew

Ingredients:

> 1 large eggplant, diced
> 1 cup dried green lentils (rinsed)
> 1 can diced tomatoes
> 1 onion, finely chopped

- ➢ 3 cloves garlic, minced
- ➢ 2 teaspoons cumin
- ➢ 1 teaspoon smoked paprika
- ➢ 4 cups vegetable broth
- ➢ Olive oil, salt, and pepper to taste

Instructions:

- ➢ In a pot, sauté onions and garlic in olive oil until softened.
- ➢ Add diced eggplant, lentils, diced tomatoes, cumin, smoked paprika, and vegetable broth.
- ➢ Simmer until lentils are cooked and the stew is thickened.
- ➢ Season with salt and pepper.

Health Benefits:

- ➢ Eggplant provides fiber and vitamins.
- ➢ Lentils offer protein and folate.
- ➢ Tomatoes add antioxidants.

Preparation Time: 35 minutes

Ingredients:

- ➢ 1 lb shrimp, peeled and deveined
- ➢ 2 mangos, diced
- ➢ 1 avocado, diced
- ➢ 1 cucumber, diced
- ➢ 1/4 cup red onion, finely chopped
- ➢ 2 tablespoons cilantro, chopped
- ➢ Lime juice, salt, and pepper to taste

Instructions:

- ➢ Grill or sauté shrimp until cooked.
- ➢ In a bowl, combine diced mangos, avocado, cucumber, red onion, and cilantro.
- ➢ Add cooked shrimp to the bowl.
- ➢ Drizzle with lime juice and season with salt and pepper.

Health Benefits:

- ➢ Shrimp provides lean protein.
- ➢ Mangos offer vitamins and antioxidants.
- ➢ Avocado adds healthy fats.

Preparation Time: 20 minutes

33: Turkey and Quinoa Stuffed Acorn Squash

Ingredients:

- 2 acorn squash, halved and seeds removed
- 1 lb ground turkey
- 1 cup cooked quinoa
- 1/2 cup dried cranberries
- 1/4 cup pecans, chopped
- 1 teaspoon cinnamon
- Olive oil, salt, and pepper to taste

Instructions:

- Preheat the oven.
- Rub acorn squash halves with olive oil, salt, and pepper.
- Roast until squash is tender.
- In a skillet, cook ground turkey until browned.
- Mix cooked turkey with quinoa, dried cranberries, pecans, and cinnamon.
- Stuff the roasted acorn squash halves with the turkey-quinoa mixture.

Health Benefits:

> Turkey provides lean protein.

> Quinoa offers complete protein.

> Acorn squash adds vitamins and fiber.

Preparation Time: 40 minutes

34: Cilantro-Lime Chicken with Avocado Salsa

Ingredients:

2 chicken breasts

1/4 cup fresh cilantro, chopped

Juice of 2 limes

2 tablespoons olive oil

1 teaspoon cumin

1 teaspoon garlic powder

Salt and pepper to taste

> **Avocado salsa:** 1 avocado, diced; 1/2 cup cherry tomatoes, halved; 1/4 cup red onion, finely chopped;

1 tablespoon fresh cilantro, chopped; Lime juice, salt, and pepper to taste

Instructions:

- ➤ In a bowl, mix chopped cilantro, lime juice, olive oil, cumin, garlic powder, salt, and pepper.
- ➤ Marinate chicken breasts in the mixture for at least 30 minutes.
- ➤ Grill or bake chicken until fully cooked.
- ➤ In a separate bowl, combine diced avocado, cherry tomatoes, red onion, cilantro, lime juice, salt, and pepper to make the salsa.
- ➤ Serve the cilantro-lime chicken topped with avocado salsa.

Health Benefits:

- ➤ Chicken provides lean protein.
- ➤ Avocado offers healthy fats.
- ➤ Cilantro and lime add fresh flavor.

Preparation Time: 35 minutes (including marination)

35: Chickpea and Vegetable Curry

Ingredients:

- ➢ 1 can chickpeas, drained and rinsed
- ➢ 1 eggplant, diced
- ➢ 1 zucchini, diced
- ➢ 1 bell pepper, sliced
- ➢ 1 onion, finely chopped
- ➢ 2 cloves garlic, minced
- ➢ 1 can coconut milk
- ➢ 2 tablespoons curry powder
- ➢ 1 tablespoon olive oil
- ➢ Basmati rice for serving

Instructions:

- ➢ In a pot, sauté onions and garlic in olive oil until softened.
- ➢ Add diced eggplant, zucchini, bell pepper, chickpeas, curry powder, and coconut milk.
- ➢ Simmer until vegetables are tender.
- ➢ Serve the curry over cooked basmati rice.

Health Benefits:

> Chickpeas offer protein and fiber.

> Eggplant provides vitamins and antioxidants.

> Coconut milk adds healthy fats.

Preparation Time: 30 minutes

36: Pecan-Crusted Tilapia

Ingredients:

> 4 tilapia fillets

> 1/2 cup pecans, finely chopped

> 2 tablespoons whole wheat flour

> 1 teaspoon paprika

> Lemon wedges for serving

> Olive oil for baking

Instructions:

> Preheat the oven.

> In a shallow dish, mix chopped pecans, whole wheat flour, and paprika.

> Coat each tilapia fillet with the pecan mixture.

> Place fillets on a baking sheet drizzled with olive oil.

> Bake until tilapia is cooked through.

> Serve with lemon wedges.

Health Benefits:

> Tilapia offers lean protein.
> Pecans provide healthy fats and antioxidants.
> Whole wheat flour adds fiber.

Preparation Time: 20 minutes

37: Sweet Potato and Turkey Skillet

Ingredients:

> 1 lb ground turkey
> 2 sweet potatoes, peeled and diced
> 1 onion, chopped
> 2 cloves garlic, minced
> 1 teaspoon cumin
> 1 teaspoon smoked paprika
> Olive oil, salt, and pepper to taste
> Fresh cilantro for garnish

Instructions:

> In a skillet, cook ground turkey until browned.
> Add diced sweet potatoes, onions, garlic, cumin, smoked paprika, olive oil, salt, and pepper.

- ➤ Cook until sweet potatoes are tender.
- ➤ Garnish with fresh cilantro before serving.

Health Benefits:

- ➤ Turkey provides lean protein.
- ➤ Sweet potatoes offer vitamins and fiber.
- ➤ Cumin and smoked paprika add flavor.

Preparation Time: 30 minutes

38: Berry and Almond Couscous Salad

Ingredients:

- ➤ 1 cup whole wheat couscous, cooked
- ➤ 1 cup mixed berries (strawberries, blueberries, raspberries)
- ➤ 1/2 cup almonds, sliced
- ➤ 1/4 cup feta cheese, crumbled
- ➤ 2 tablespoons balsamic vinaigrette dressing
- ➤ Fresh mint leaves for garnish

Instructions:

- ➤ In a bowl, combine cooked couscous, mixed berries, sliced almonds, and crumbled feta cheese.
- ➤ Drizzle with balsamic vinaigrette dressing.

> Toss gently and garnish with fresh mint leaves.

Health Benefits:

> Whole wheat couscous provides complex carbohydrates.
> Berries offer antioxidants.
> Almonds add healthy fats.

Preparation Time: 15 minutes

39: Black Bean and Corn Salsa

Ingredients:

> 1 can black beans, drained and rinsed
> 1 cup corn kernels (fresh or frozen)
> 1 red bell pepper, diced
> 1/4 cup red onion, finely chopped
> 1 jalapeño, seeded and minced
> 2 tablespoons cilantro, chopped
> Juice of 2 limes
> Salt and pepper to taste

Instructions:

- In a bowl, combine black beans, corn, diced red bell pepper, red onion, jalapeño, cilantro, lime juice, salt, and pepper.
- Mix well and refrigerate for at least 30 minutes.
- Serve as a refreshing salsa with whole grain tortilla chips or as a topping for grilled chicken or fish.

Health Benefits:

- Black beans offer protein and fiber.
- Corn provides vitamins and antioxidants.
- Bell pepper adds vitamins and flavor.

Preparation Time: 15 minutes

40: Lemon Garlic Shrimp with Quinoa

Ingredients:

- 1 lb shrimp, peeled and deveined
- 1 cup quinoa, cooked
- 3 cloves garlic, minced
- Zest and juice of 2 lemons
- 2 tablespoons olive oil
- Fresh parsley for garnish
- Salt and pepper to taste

Instructions:

> - In a pan, sauté minced garlic in olive oil until fragrant.
> - Add shrimp and cook until pink and opaque.
> - Stir in lemon zest and juice.
> - Serve the lemon garlic shrimp over cooked quinoa.
> - Garnish with fresh parsley.

Health Benefits:

> - Shrimp provides lean protein.
> - Quinoa offers complete protein.
> - Lemon and garlic add flavor.

Preparation Time: 20 minutes

CONCLUSION

The Male Fertility Cookbook serves as a comprehensive guide to nourishing both body and fertility. Focused on optimizing nutritional intake, these recipes are thoughtfully crafted to support male reproductive health, providing a delicious and practical way to embrace a fertility-conscious lifestyle.

As we've explored a variety of ingredients and culinary techniques, it becomes evident that promoting fertility extends beyond mere sustenance – it's about embracing a flavorful, wholesome approach to nourishment.

Each recipe not only tantalizes the taste buds but also harnesses the power of nutrients known for their positive impact on male reproductive function.

The journey through the Male Fertility Cookbook has been more than a culinary exploration; it's an investment in well-being, vitality, and the pursuit of a healthier future.

By incorporating these recipes into your daily routine, you're not only savoring delightful dishes but also taking proactive steps toward enhancing fertility.

Remember, the key to success lies not just in the ingredients, but in the consistency of mindful choices.

May this cookbook inspire you to embark on a nourishing journey that not only delights your palate but also contributes to the overall well-being of your reproductive health.

Embrace these recipes, cultivate a lifestyle that supports fertility, and savor the joy of taking charge of your health in every delicious bite.

Here's to a future filled with flavor, health, and the promise of new beginnings!